FIX YOUR FEET

USING THE

PILATES METHOD

Kathryn Ross-Nash

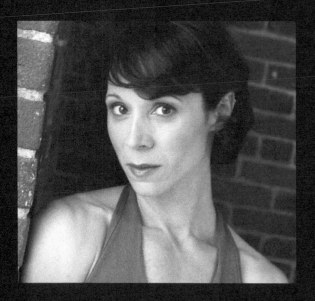

FIX YOUR FEET

Written by world renown Pilates Instructor. Kathryn Ross-Nash takes you through the exercises she was given by her mentor, Romana Kryzanowska, after a horrible ankle injury. Not only did they aid in the recuperation of the ankle, but also helped shrink bunions from 25 plus years of ballet.

Since then, Kathryn has used this method to aid in the rehabilitation of many feet - including her own daughter. The secret of Joe Pilates is out. Now you an fix your feet and return a bounce to your step.

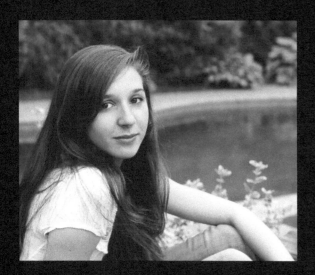

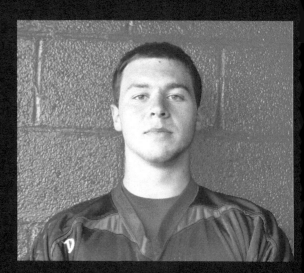

Photo's by Zoe Ross-Nash and Zachary Cosmo Ross-Nash
Written and Demonstrated by Kathryn Ross-Nash

ABOUT THE AUTHOR

Kathryn began her Pilates training in 1980. She has had the privilege to be trained by Romana Kryzanowska, Kathy Grant, Sari Mejo Santos, Jay Grime and Edwina Fontaine and all first generation teachers. She is a level 2 Teacher Trainer for Romana's Certification Program. She holds certification through Romana's Pilates, The Pilates Studio, The Authentic Pilates Guild, AFTA, IFFA and is a Guild Certified Feldenkrais Practitioner. Kathryn was a principle dancer for ten years with Ballet Hispanico of NY and often returns to restage ballets. She also holds a second degree black belt in Te Kwon Do and an undefeated AAU sparring record.

Kathryn worked side by side with Romana for many years. She has demonstrated the advanced work for her at workshops and seminars throughout the US. She is the only woman to demonstrate on both the Romana's Pilates DVD's and the Legacy Series. Romana is quoted about Ms. Ross-Nash that her work is like ice cream and that she is one of her best, her "star of stars". Kathryn was also hand picked by Romana to sit at her right hand as the founding vice-president of The Authentic Pilates Guild.

Ms. Ross-Nash was also a feature instructor in the premiere issue of Pilates Style Magazine, infomercial and many other Pilates Style issues. Kathryn was invited to be one of the three premiere writers for Pilates Style International Blog. She is often a quoted expert and her advise on the method is sought after world wide.

Know throughout the industry for her purity and devotion to the work, her list of students include many in the TV, movie, broadway, professional athletes, dancers and music industry. She was invited as the first instructor to train the dancers of the Vaganova School in St Petersburgh, Russia. Ross-Nash continues to train teachers throughout the world. "My favorite thing in the world is to be able to teach the work I believe in so strongly" says Ross-Nash, "as my teacher so generously gave to me".

TABLE OF CONTENTS

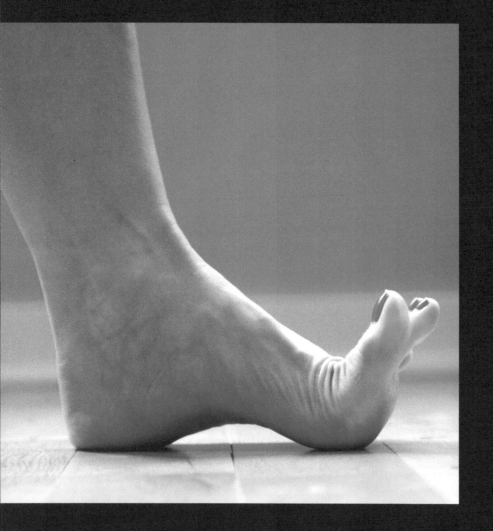

TOWEL

PENCIL

WAVE

ARCH

MARBLES

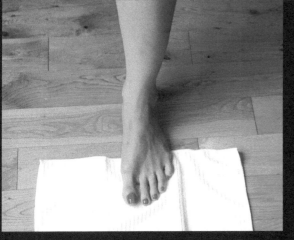

TOWEL

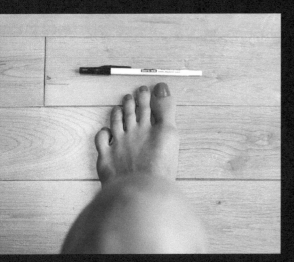

PENCIL

TOOLS NEEDED

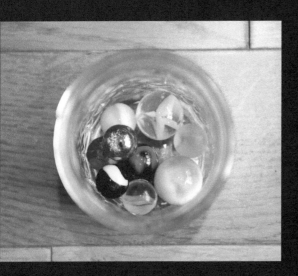

MARBLES & JAR

BODY POSITION OPTIONS

1. Sitting with Legs Bent - hands by hips

2. Sitting with Legs Straight . hands by hips

3. Standing with Two Straight Legs

4. Standing, Front Leg Bent, Back Leg Straight

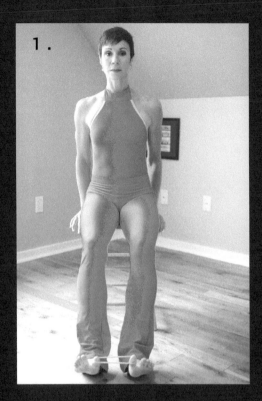
1.

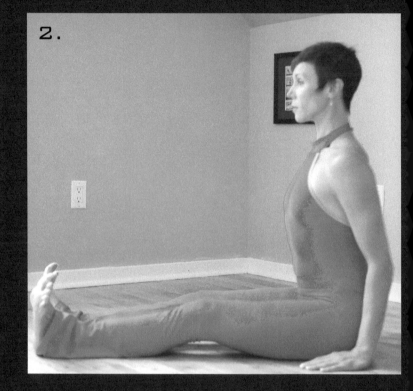
2.

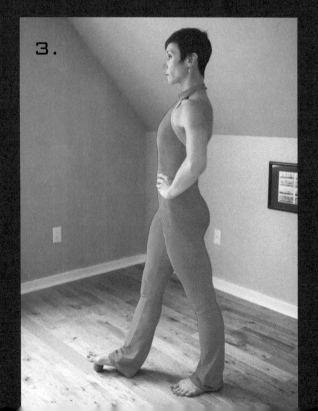
3.

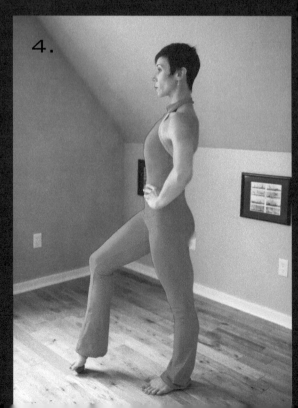
4.

5.

ARM OPTIONS

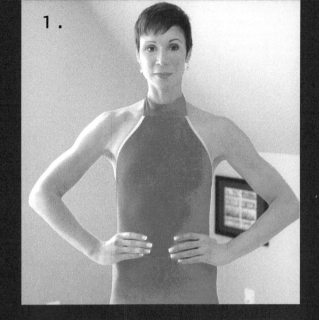

1. Hand On Hips - Helps find alignment.

2. Out to Side - Helps with balance.

3. Crossed in Front Shoulder Height - increased balance needed.

4 Hand on Hand Behind the Head - opens chest and challenges stability.

Note: If balance is an issue - can be done holding a ballet barre or a chair.

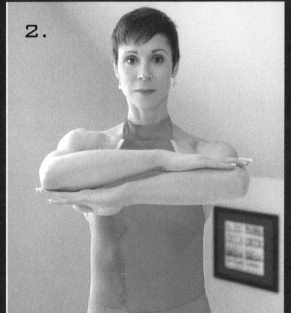

Whenever you are working, remember to engage your core by pulling your stomach in and up to support your spine. Be very careful not to arch your back. Imagine there is a wall behind you and your core is pressing your spine in and up the imaginary wall.

Also, be aware that your hips and shoulders are parallel to each other with equal distance from rib to hip on both sides of your body. I recommend using a mirror when working.

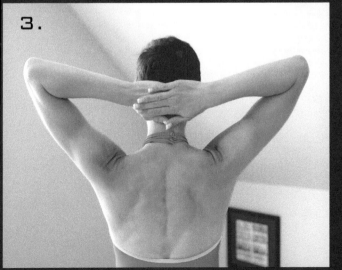

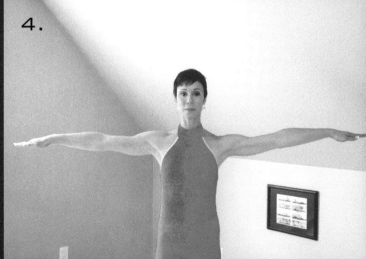

TOWEL . PENCIL . WAVE . ARCH

Choose an Arm Position and a Body Position standing (1) or sitting with legs bent at a 90 degree angle hands by hips (2). The Arm Positions are listed in the order of difficulty from easiest to most difficult. All the these exercises may be performed while holding onto a chair or barre for balance. Try to build your strength and increase your balance over time with practice.

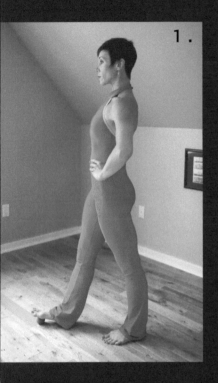

1.

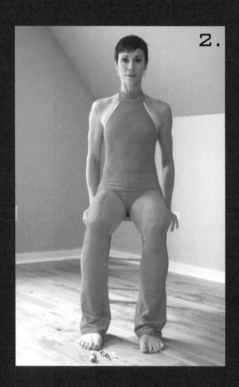

2.

****

It is very important to engage your core and have correct alignment when doing these exercises. Do not sacrifice using your stomach and keeping the hips and shoulders square when trying to gather the towel. The alignment of your body will effect the alignment of your feet. Try not to move your body when doing all these exercises. In other words, isolate the movement of the foot, ankle, knee and hip. Stabilize your body by creating length in your spine. I like to think of a two directional pull and a strong center. The crown of my head reaches toward the ceiling and my tailbone reaches to the floor. My core engages too for a girdle of strength around my middle, supporting my spine.

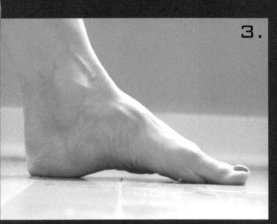

3.

Note: Very important! When working be sure that the arch of your foot is lifted off the floor. Three points touch- ball big toe, ball little toe and heel of foot. (3)

Choosing *a body and arm position:* When choosing an arm position think about what suits you best. The first thing to always check, when working, is that *your core is engaged.* The next thing to check is that your **hips and shoulders** are in alignment. This is why I recommend holding onto a chair or barre first and then using the *hands on hips position (1.).* This position helps you see and feel the alignment of your body.

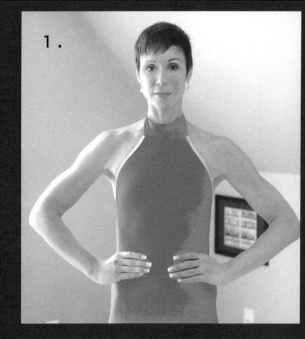

In Pilates, the core is referred to as the *Powerhouse or Girdle of Strength* (as I prefer). The Girdle of Strength is created by engaging the abdominal muscle and lifting them in and up. This action creates space and support in the spine. To find this action you can stand with your back against the wall with your knees bent. Press your entire spine against the wall by pulling your core in and up. Try to keep the ribcage down and isolate the stomach muscles. I think about creating a two way street with a strong intersection. My powerhouse being the intersection and my head lifting up through the ceiling and my tailbone reaching down for the floor. The shoulders and hips facing one direction and forming parallel lines is referred to as the Box in Pilates. You always want to be sure that your box is square.This helps to promote healthy spinal alignment. I call these rules of working, the Rules of Engagement. Powerhouse first, Box second, Exercise third. Use this guideline throughout the book.

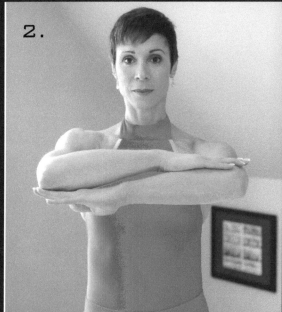

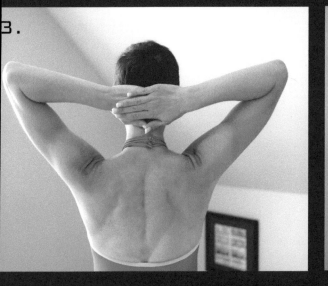

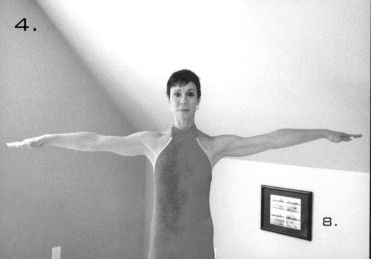

THE TOWEL

develops arch & increases circulation

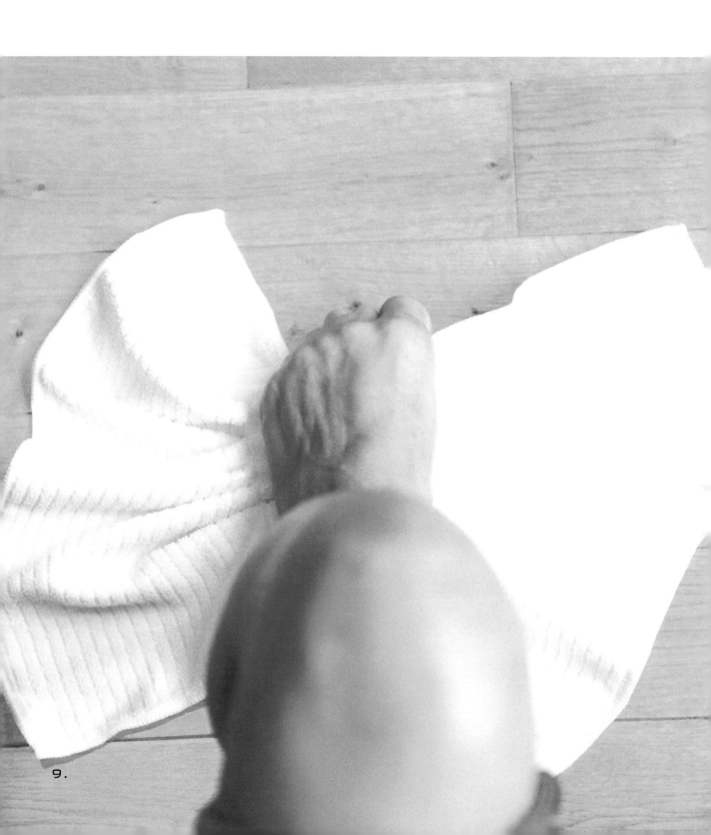

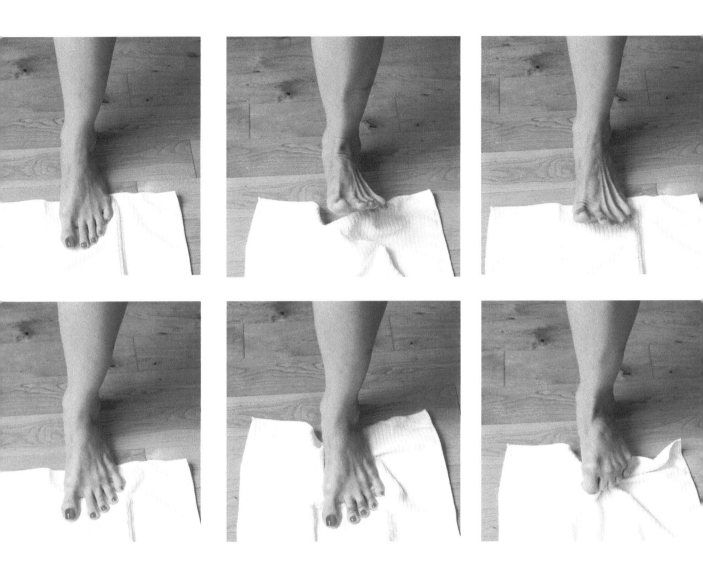

1. Spread a small hand towel out and have your box square. Keep your foot in a line with your ankle, knee and hip.
2. Engage your core and flex your foot keeping your heel on the floor.
3. Flex the foot lifting the toes evenly.
4. Spread your toes and keeping them straight, place them on the towel.
5. Grab the towel with spread toes and PULL the towel in towards your heel. Be sure to use all your toes.
6. Repeat until towel is curled all the way in.
7. Reverse the action and PUSH the towel out and away.
8. Repeat three to five times with each foot, then both feet at the same time.

Note: If you have a weaker foot, repeat the exercise an extra time with that foot.

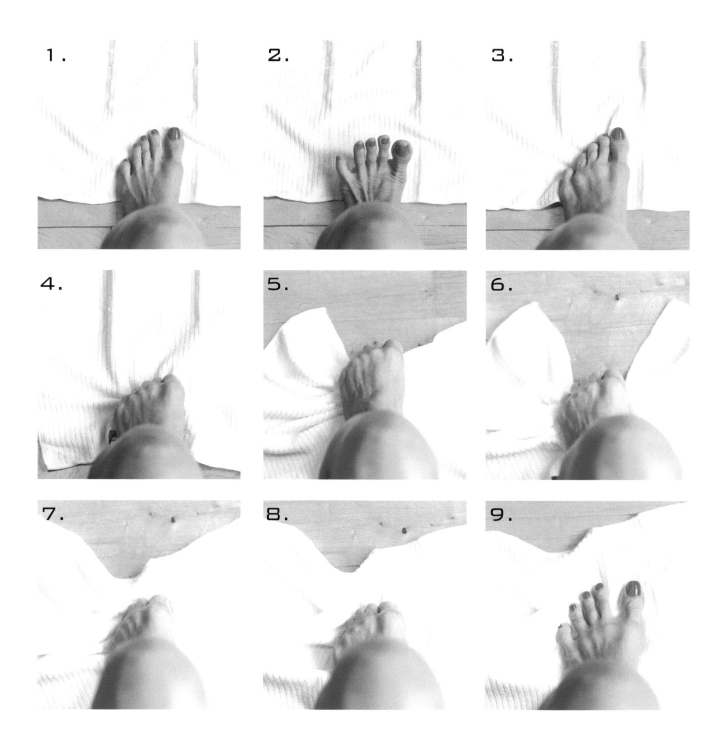

1. 2. 3.
4. 5. 6.
7. 8. 9.

I prefer sitting with knees over ankles first. It makes it easier to see the alignment of the hip, knee, ankle and toes.

Photos one through six demonstrate pulling the towel in.
Photos seven through nine show pushing the towel out.

THE PENCIL

improves motor skills of the foot
develops arch & increases circulation

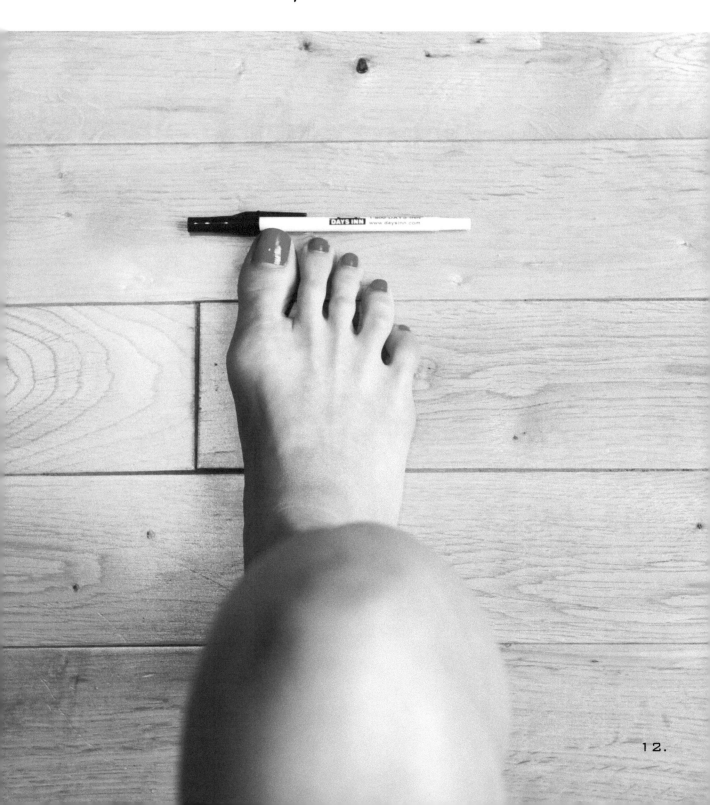

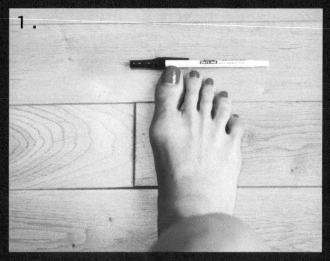
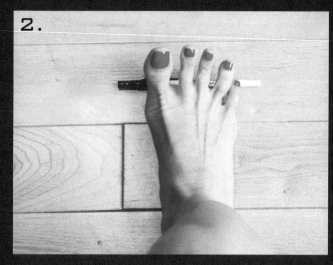
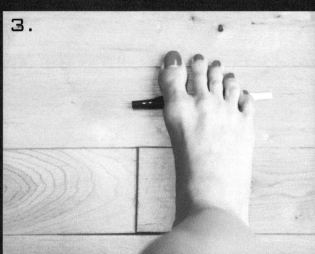
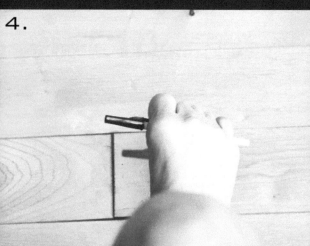

Use the same *body and arm position* as the *Towel*.

1. Line toes, ankle, knee and hip up with pencil/pen.

2. Lift toes and flex the toes back and over the pen.
   Try to keep your heel on the floor to increase difficulty and preserve alignment.

3. Spread ALL toes over the pencil/pen.

4. Grasp pencil with ALL toes and lift the pencil. Hold for three to five counts.

5. Repeat three to five times each foot.

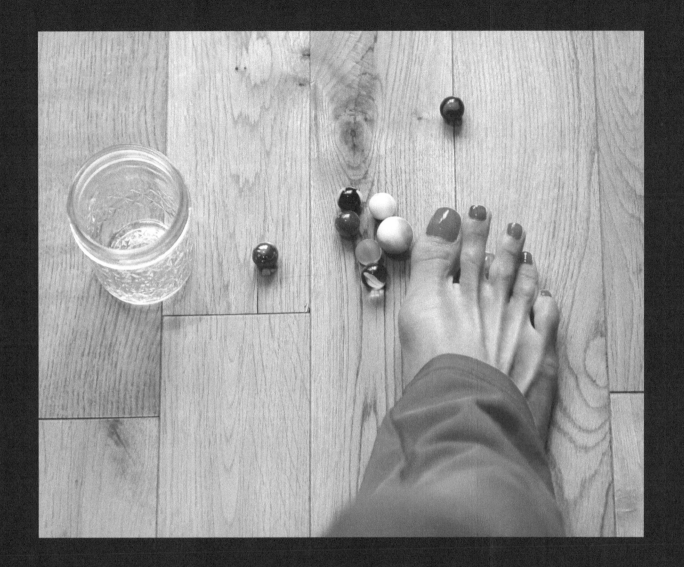

THE MARBLES

increases dexterity and balance
improves motor function and co-ordination

BODY AND ARM
POSITION OPTIONS

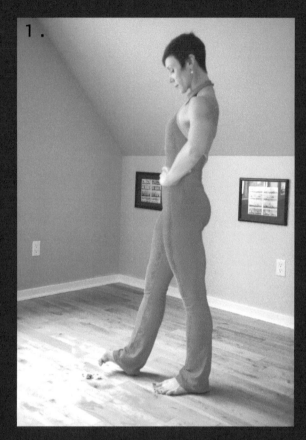

1.

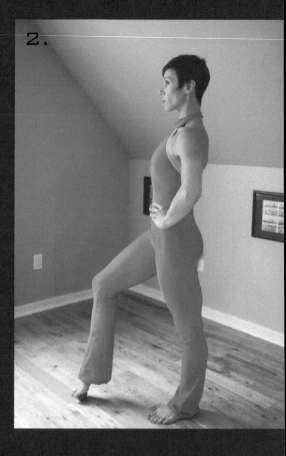

2.

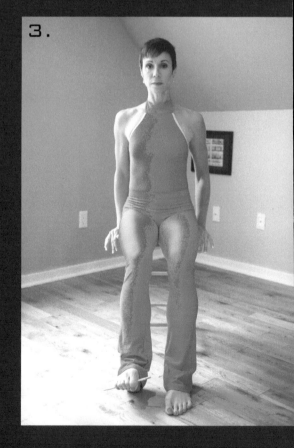

3.

Choose from:

Standing Straight Leg (1)

Standing with Front Leg Bent (2)

Sitting with Knees Bent (3)

Choose whatever arm
position suits you best.

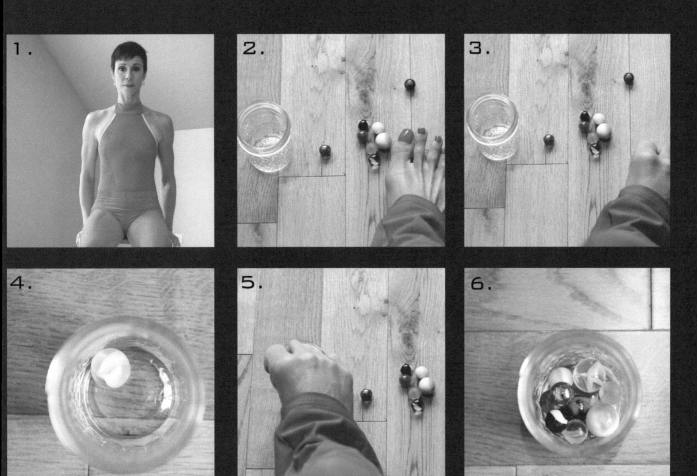

1. Choose body and arm position

2. Spread ten marbles on the floor next to a jar.

3. Pick up marbles with one foot and place them in the jar. Repeat five marbles each foot.

4. Challenge yourself and try to pick up one marble at a time with each individual toe.
   Begin with the largest to to the smallest toe. Each time placing the marble in the jar.

T H E

W A V E

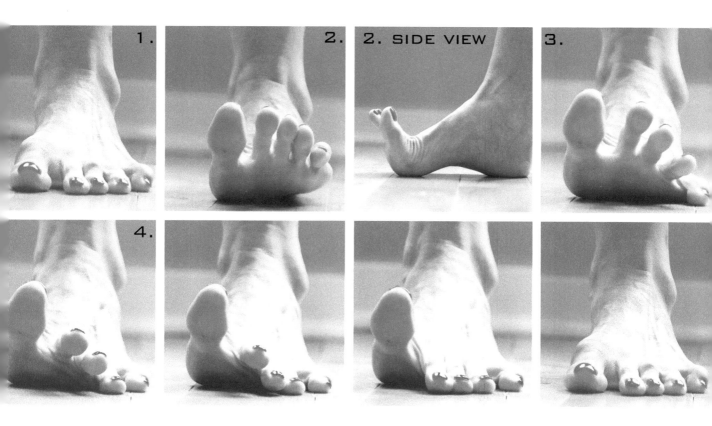

1. Choose an **Arm Position** and a **Body Position** standing or sitting with legs bent at a 90 degree angle.

   Be sure that the **Girdle of Strength** is engaged and the **Box is square**.
   Make sure the center of your foot lines up with your ankle, knee and hip.

2. Flex your toes back in a straight line. Be careful not to rock to either side of the foot.

3. Place ONLY the pinky toe on the ground and keep all other toes lifted.

4. Repeat this action with the second toe, the third, forth and fifth.
   Be sure to articulate the movement and only let one toe touch to join the others already down.

5. Repeat this five to eight times with one foot then the other.
   If you have a weaker foot do that foot first, then the other foot and then repeat the weaker foot.

Note: Once you have mastered this, reverse the action or do two feet at one time!   1 8.

CHALLENGE YOURSELF
TRY TWO FEET AT ONCE

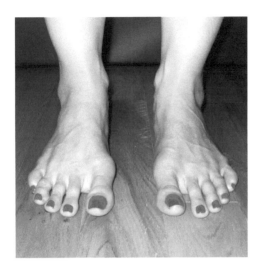 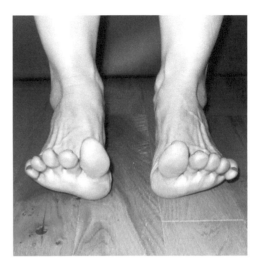

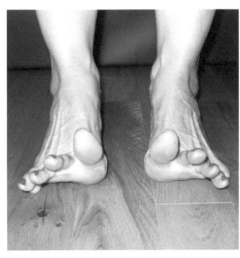 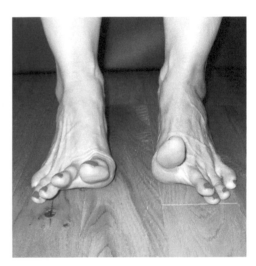

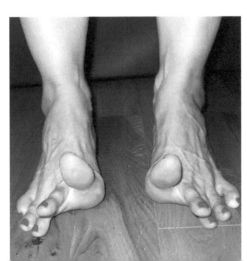 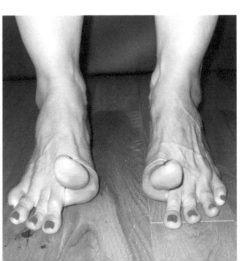

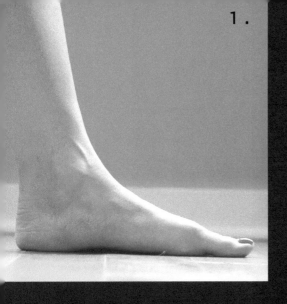

THE ARCH

LIFTS ARCHES & FIGHTS PLANTAR FASCIITIS

1. Choose an **Arm Position and a Body Position** standing or sitting with legs bent at a 90 degree angle. Be sure that the **Girdle of Strength** is engaged and the **box is square**. Make sure the center of your foot lines up with your ankle, knee and hip. Foot flat on the ground.

2. Flex toes up and hold for three to five counts. Return to flat.

3. Scoop arch of foot off the ground - dragging toes. Hold for three to five counts.

4. Curl arch deeper to lift ball of foot off the ground as well. Hold for three to five counts.

5. Return to flat and repeat five to eight times with the same foot. Repeat with the other foot. If there is a weaker foot, do the exercise on the weaker foot, then the stronger foot and repeat on the weaker foot.

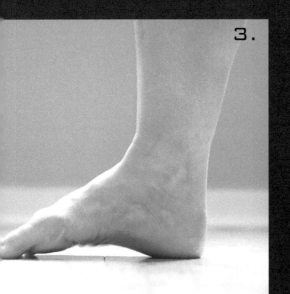

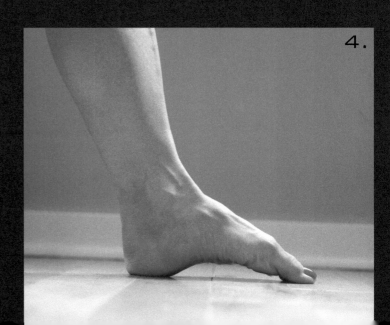

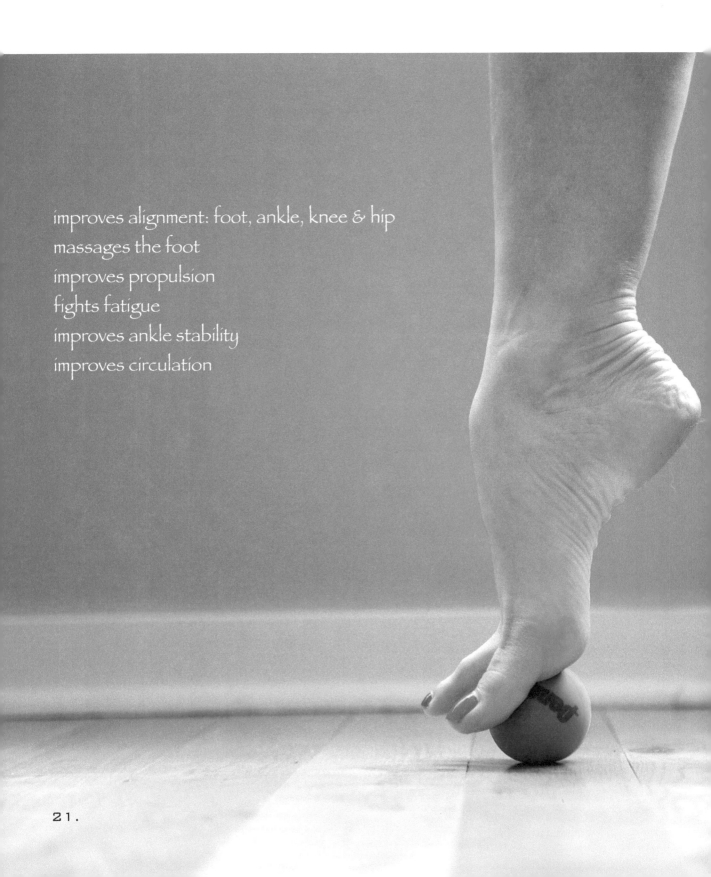

improves alignment: foot, ankle, knee & hip
massages the foot
improves propulsion
fights fatigue
improves ankle stability
improves circulation

TOOLS NEEDED

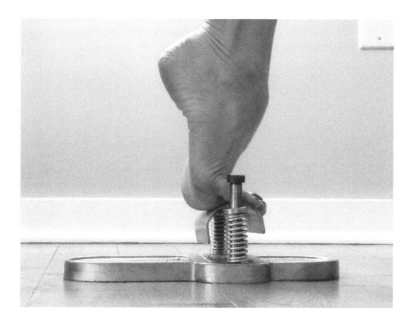

GRATZ FOOT CORRECTOR

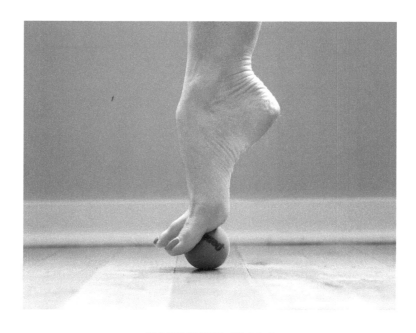

RUBBER BALL

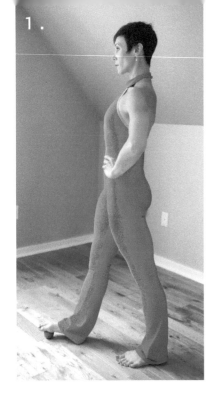
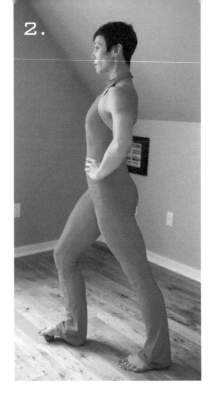
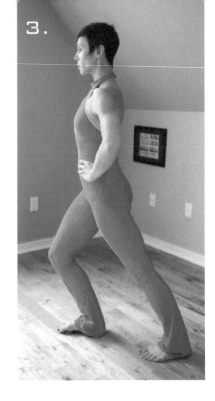

BODY POSITION OPTIONS

1. Two Straight Legs: Ankle Isolation
   Move only the ankle - for ankle strength
   and stability. Helps to increase propulsion.

2. Front Leg Bent: Ankle Isolation
   Move only the ankle - for ankle strength
   and alignment.

3. Front Leg Bent Lunge: Weight Shift
   Move the body, using the buttocks,
   hip and ankle.

4. High Heel: Hip Isolation or Shift
   Press pedal from the hip to strengthen
   hip or shift weight for ankle stability.

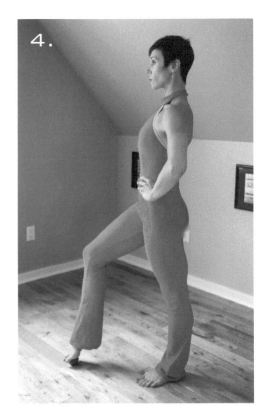

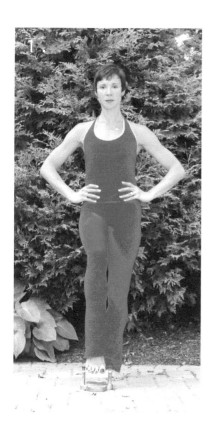

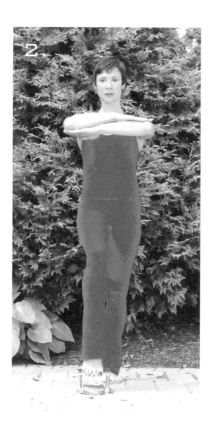

1. Hand On Hips -
   Helps find alignment.

2. Crossed in Front
   Shoulder Height -
   increased balance
   needed.

3. Out to Side -
   Helps with balance.

4. Hand on Hand
   Behind the Head -
   opens chest and
   challenges stability.

ARM OPTIONS

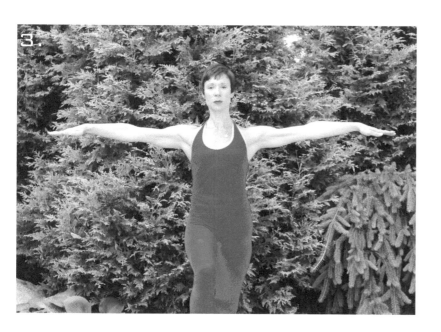

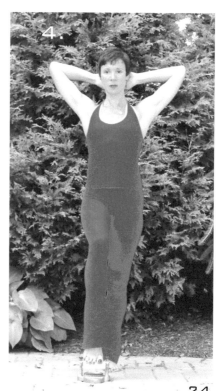

Note: If balance is an issue –
can be done holding a ballet barre or a chair.

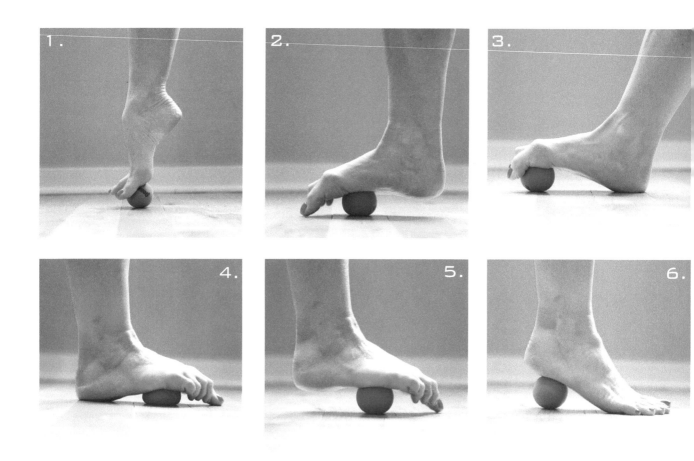

FOOT POSITION
BALL OF THE FOOT

1. Heel up (High Heel) - Ankle stability and hip and buttocks strengthening
2. Heel Level - Ankle stability and control
3. Heel Down - Achilles stretch
4. Ball of the foot - Heel down
5. Arch of the foot - Heel level
6. Heel of the foot

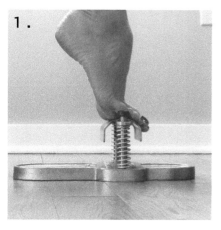
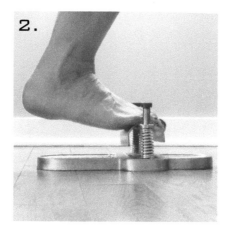
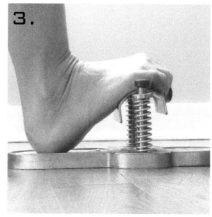
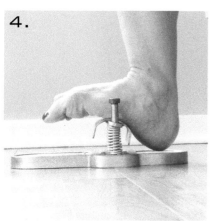
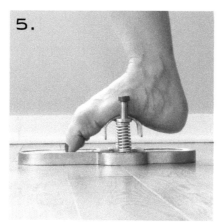
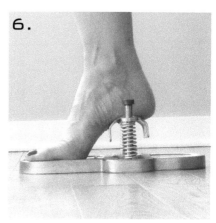

FOOT POSITION
FOOT CORRECTOR

1. Arch of Foot - Heel Down - Achilles stretch
2. Arch of the Foot - Heel Up - Achilles stretch and ankle stretch
3. Heel of Foot - Ankle stability and leg strength
4. Ball of the foot - Heel down
5. Arch of the foot - Heel level
6. Heel of the foot

PRESSING OPTIONS

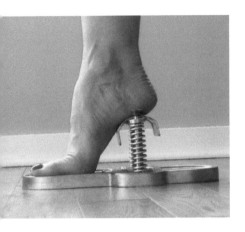 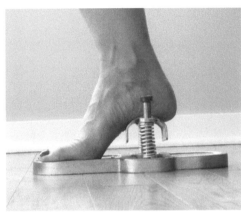 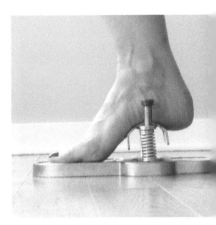

When pressing begin by choosing a **foot position** and an **arm position** that suits your needs and challenges your ability. They are listed in the order of difficulty. After choosing **foot and arm position**, begin by simply pressing and releasing the pedal (ball).

Be sure that each movement comes from your **core and that your shoulders and hips remain square** throughout. Watch the pedal (ball) and be sure that it lowers and lifts evenly. After this is mastered, build yourself by using the press options listed in each **foot position and arm position**. Also, build your strength by increasing the time you hold the press in each position and the number of times you press the pedal (ball).

PRESSING VARIATIONS

VARIATIONS

1. Press and Release

2. Press Half Way and Release

3. Press Fully and Release

4. Press Half Way, Hold and Release

5. Press Fully, Hold and Release

6. Press Half Way, Hold, Press Fully,
   Hold and Release

7. Press Half Way, Hold, Press Fully, Hold,
   Release Half Way, Hold and Release

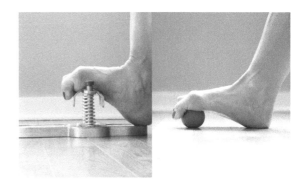

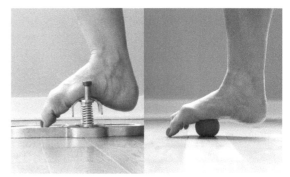

COUNTS

Begin with the first variation:

Press 3 counts & release 3 counts - 5x's

Build to an 8 count - press & 8 count and

release - 5x's

Then increase the repetitions to 10.

Repeat this process with each Pressing

Option.

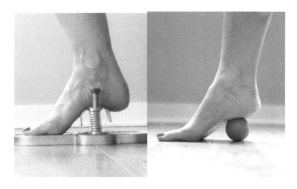

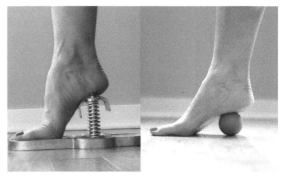

Note: These Pressing Options are meant to be done
separately, not all together.
An example of a combination is: Ball of the Foot (Foot Position)
- 2 Straight Legs (Body Position) - Pressing Option 1 (Pressing Option)
- Hands on Hips (Arm Position)
Repeat Pressing Option on the Arch and then the Heel. Followed by the Massage.

THE MASSAGE

1. Begin in **Position 3** with the back leg straight and the front leg bent.

2. **Ball of the foot** is on pedal(ball) with heel down.

3. **Shift weight** on to ball of foot to compress pedal (ball).

4. **Slide foot** over pedal(ball) with even pressure. Do not let pedal shift side to side or rise and fall.

5. **Slide** through the **arch** with **heel down**, **arch** with **heel up** & onto the **heel**. Reverse the action to return to start position.

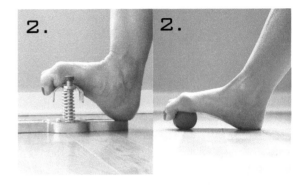

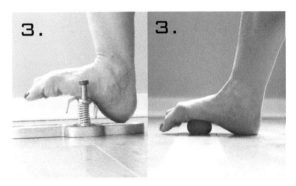

Note: Be sure to curl the toes around the pedal as you begin to slide.

Choose Arm Position to suit and challenge you. Remember this can be done using a barre or chair for support. Be sure to work from your core throughout the exercise and to keep hips and shoulders square (facing forward).

This is always a great way to end the Foot Corrector (ball) work.

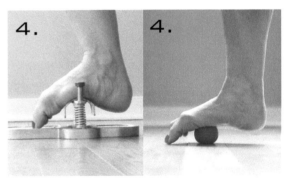

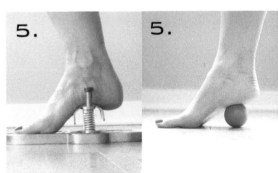

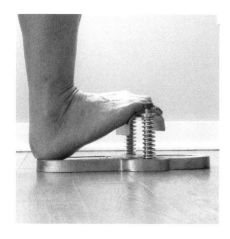 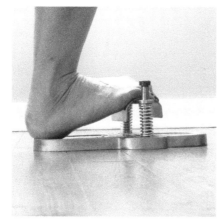 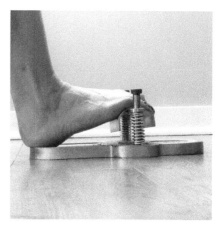

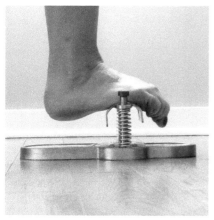 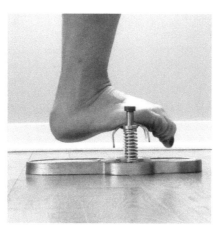 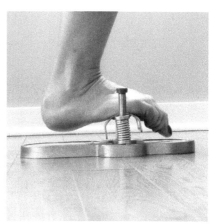

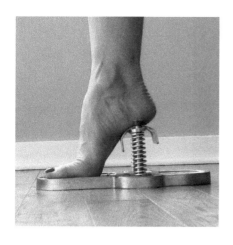 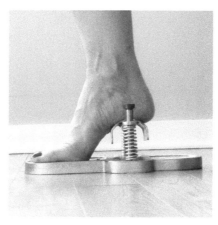 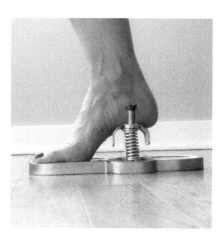

THE TOE STRETCHER
& THE ELASTIC BAND

The Bunion Fixer!

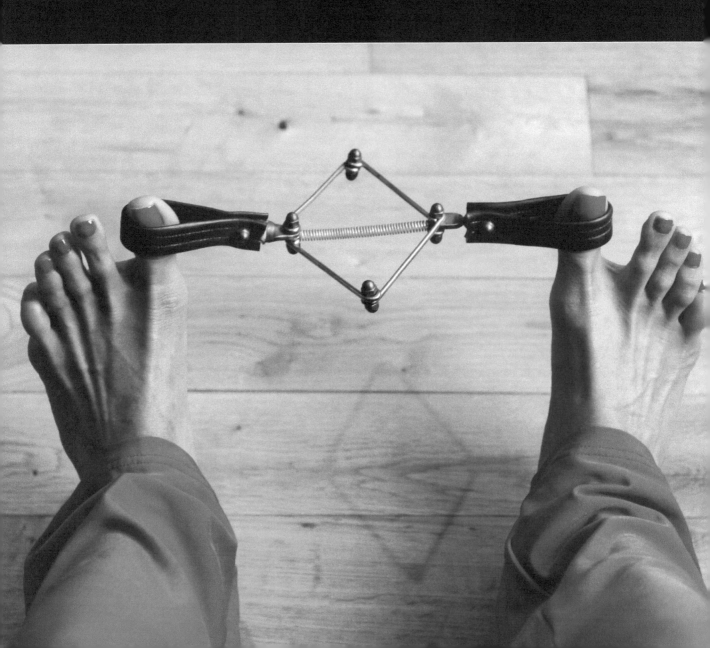

TOOLS NEEDED

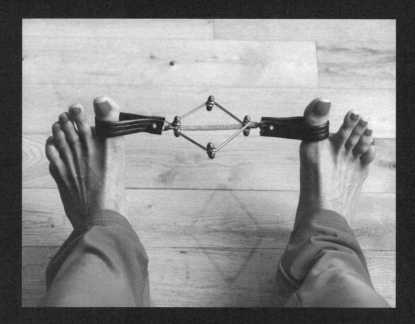

GRATZ PILATES TOE STRETCHER

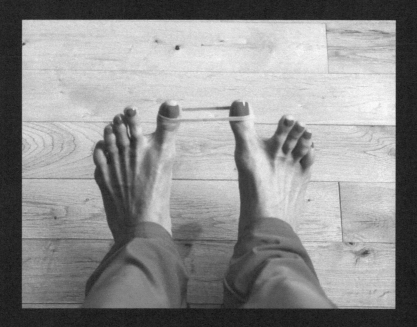

THICK ELASTIC BAND
like used on a head of broccoli

BODY POSITION OPTIONS

Choose from either *Sitting Upright* with legs bent at a 90 degree angle or **Sitting** with the legs out stretched. Whatever position you choose be sure that you are sitting directly on your **sitz** bones, not behind. Once again, imagine there is a wall behind you and your entire spine is against it. You can begin by doing this exercise with your back against a wall if it helps you from rocking back. Just be careful not to hyper-extend your knees. Place your hands by your hips and roll your shoulders back to open your chest. Be sure to keep your rib cage down and the *powerhouse engaged* with *hips and shoulders square*. Remember to include your neck in your alignment.

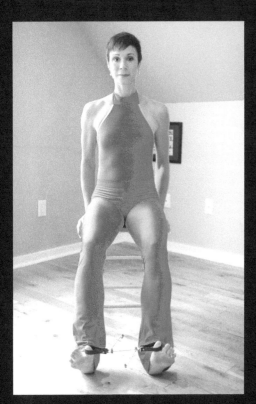
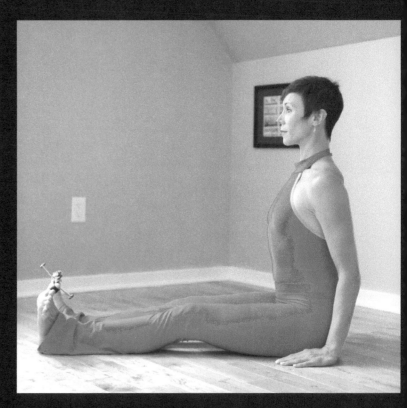

When *sitting with legs long*, your feet can be parallel and apart or with heels together. In either position be sure that the movement begins from the *powerhouse* without disturbing the *box*. The rotation of the movement comes from inside the hip, not the ankle. The Ankle remains stable throughout. This builds stability in the alignment. Also imagine the two way street when moving. With each action, feel longer and taller.

A variation used for ankle flexibility would be to add a rotation of the ankle to the original hip rotation. This is usually reserved for dancers.

STRETCHER OR
ELASTIC POSITION OPTIONS

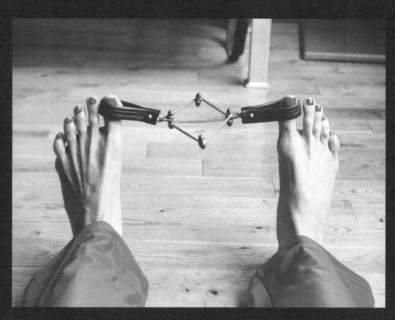

Place the Stretcher or Band up high on the first joint.

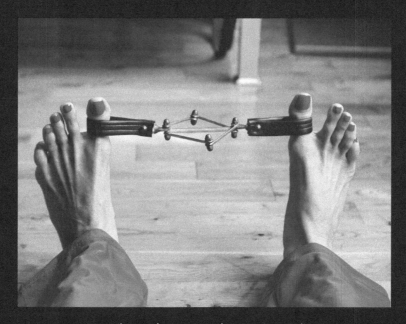

Place the Stretcher or Band
down low toward the base of the toe.

Choose the easiest position for your toes first. Everyone is different...

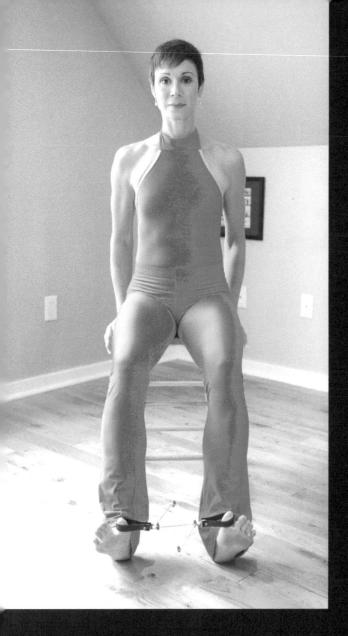

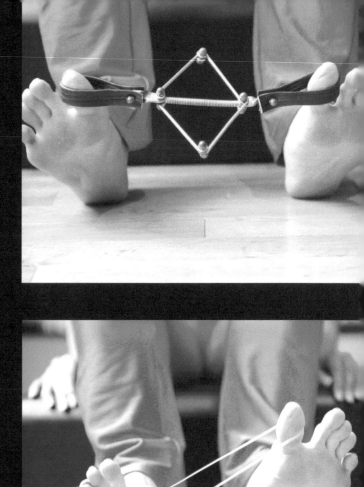

Be sure when seated with legs bent that you move from your hip and do not twist your knee. If a 90 degree angle of the knee is too great for either knee or the hip, extend knee to a comfortable position.

THE SIMPLE TOE STRETCH

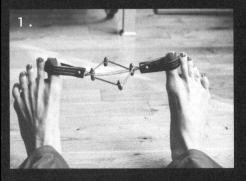

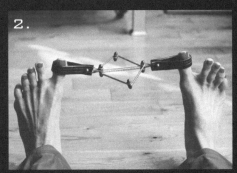

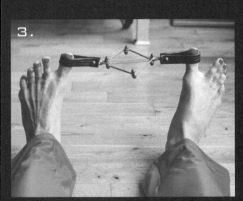

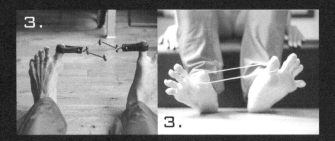

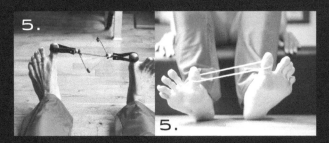

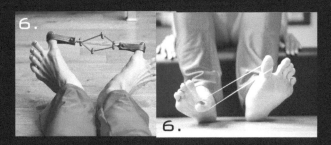

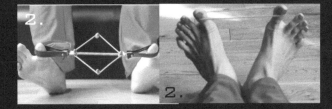

Maintain a lifted seated position if you are sitting.
Tendency is to sink or slouch as you move.

1. Choose sitting, arm and toe stretcher/elastic position.
2. Engage Stretcher by engaging the core and rotating from the hips. You should feel your buttocks working!!
3. Once spring on Stretcher or elastic is engaged, increase the pull on the right side by rotating the right leg out more.
4. Hold 3-5 count and repeat 5-8 times. Releasing fully between each pull.
5. Repeat action pulling the toe up or toward you.
6. Repeat action pushing the toe down or away from you.
7. Repeat all the Stretches using both feet at the same time. Rotating from both hips equally and maintain the alignment with your shoulders and hips.

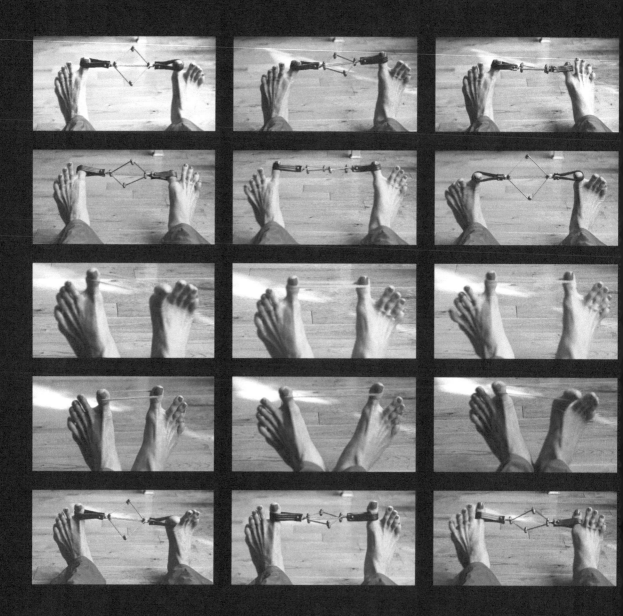

1. SINGLE TOE CIRCLES:

Keeping one toe and foot steady, engage the spring (elastic) press toe down (away) and hold for 3-5 counts.

- keep tension and move toe to the side
- hold 3-5 counts then pull toe up (toward you) hold 3-5 counts
- repeat 5-8 times
- reverse action

2. SINGLE TOE 1/4 CIRCLES:

Use this if one motion is more difficult to do.

- Keep one toe and foot steady
- engage the spring (elastic) press the toe down
- hold 3-5 counts
- keep tension and move to the side
- keep tension and return down
- release tension and repeat 5-8 times
- reverse action

3. SINGLE TOE SEMI-CIRCLES

- Keep one toe and foot steady
- engage spring (elastic)
- press down (away)
- keep tension, move side and up
- release tension and repeat 3-5 times
- reverse, press up, side, down

This can be done without release: engage spring, press down, side, up, side down, release 3-5 times.

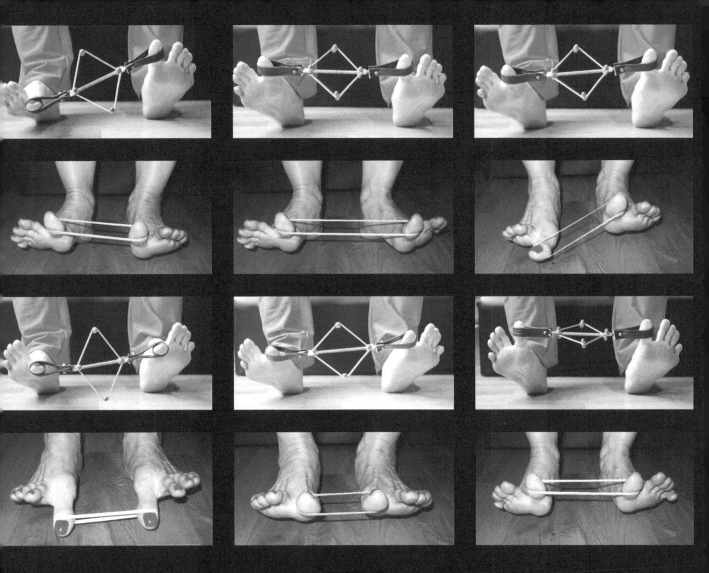

DOUBLE TOE STRETCH

All single toe stretches can and should be built up to be done with two feet at the same time. Another option for weaker side is to do double toe exercises and end with single toe on weaker side. You can also try all of the exercises with both the first and second toe in the stretcher (elastic band) and remember if there is a weaker or tighter side to begin and end with that side.

www.ingramcontent.com/pod-product-compliance
Lightning Source LLC
LaVergne TN
LVHW071754110225
803331LV00027B/31

* 9 7 8 1 4 5 0 7 4 0 8 0 7 *